Love Your Body, Change Your Life

Book Two

EMMA WRIGHT

DEDICATION

For Mum

CONTENTS

GRATITUDE

I couldn't have chosen a creative career without my sister, who leads by example and inspires me to accomplish things that matter. My brother and sister-in-law who make a living from their creativity and always see the best in people. Tom who made me promise to keep going and Suzie who relentlessly demonstrates what following a dream requires.

Thanks to my mothers, all four of you, in order of appearance: Mum, for passing on an expansive love of reading and for calling me a writer way before I could see that gift in myself; Faysie, for being the ears and wisdom I needed when life went wonky; Ellie, for being the role model I always wanted; Ann for being a living example of unconditional love.

Dad for encouraging me to follow my heart, always, regardless of…anything.

My creative friends; my mummy friends who kept (and still keep) me sane when the grenade that is children exploded into my life; my long-time friends who lent an ear, gave a hug, pulled out a stern sort-yourself-out when necessary. Hugs to you all.

Everyone else who touched my life, inspired me, allowed me to create and, of course, bought my work.

Caroline for editing that not only made my words sparkle, but brought heart, generosity, love and guidance. Deeply humbled to have worked with you.

All of you darling people who proof-read, beta-read, gave me feed-back; Jo in particular. So lucky to have you on my court.

Last, in no way least (in fact, most), my family: my immediate one, G (I'm so grateful for the life we are creating) and our two darlings (seriously, love like I've never known); and my wider scrambling messy fabulous whanau (Maori for; extended family including blood relatives and extra close friends). You know who you are.

Introduction

To The Series

"I'm thankful for my struggle

because without it

I wouldn't have stumbled across my strength"

~ *Alex Elle*

This series is best read in the order it is written; *Book One*, then *Book Two*, etc. That said, reading it out of order, totally works too. Each book can stand on its own. So, if you have come to this one first, feel free to jump right in.

After all, this book is about acceptance, and as you'll soon discover, there has never been a better time to start accepting. Acceptance for me changed everything. When I was neck deep in the binge/purge cycle of hell, I used to think bulimia and its constant companion — hatred of my physical body — was the worst thing ever; the shame of it.

Seriously, who eats like that and then makes herself sick? And worse still, doesn't stop? I knew I should. For my teeth, if nothing else. And yet, I couldn't. The bliss that eating gave me was a powerful force. A release. The take-me-away-from-the-hideousness-of-the-relentless-self-hatred was strong. I couldn't willpower myself out of it. Nor psychotherapy my way through it. I couldn't rationalize, strategize, nor kid myself from doing it. Even while it almost killed me.

And yet, today, I'll tell anyone my experience has been a blessing. That didn't happen overnight. It took almost ten years from finally stopping (I'm forty-seven now) to be able to say: Every drop of hideousness was worth something. I wouldn't give back one binge, one thought of self-hatred, one ounce of shame. Each step brought me here, and I'm good with it. Today, food doesn't dominate me, I live a fulfilling creative life, and, perhaps best of all I can laugh at myself and feel deeply connected to others.

If you are at the end of your tether with food, I want you to know: There is a way out. Living a free and abundant life, like you've always wanted, is possible. I'm here to show you how.

Let's dive straight into getting your head around the power of acceptance.

My recovery started in a small room in LA where I reached the end of my rope. My version of bottoming out was realizing I was trying the same things (diets, fasts, health regimes, exercise, willpower, purging) again and again and again to change the way I ate (and the size of my body), and those things weren't ever going to work. And at the very same time, I got that the goal I'd been chasing (a skinny little minx of a body) was never going to give me what I really wanted anyway. That false promise sold to us all — that being a certain weight, shape and size came crashing down, house of cards fashion. If being skinny isn't going to get me what I really want, what on the God-given earth is?

So there it was and there I was, feeling lost and bewildered. All I could do was acknowledge that it was time to take an entirely new approach. I decided then and there to open my arms and welcome in the beast. That included the bone scary decision to stop trying to stop; stop trying to fix myself like I was broken. I would turn toward accepting myself in the present (with all my shortcomings, quirks, defects, and wobbly bits) instead of holding out for some day in the future when I was more deserving.

At first, the task of learning to love and accept every inch of 'me'— including bulimia — looked about as possible as understanding Stephen Hawking's theories. I didn't know if I was up to it. And yet, it occurred to me, this might be the only chance I get to have the life I really wanted — the one I ached for — which made me willing. I decided to take small steps, to point myself in the direction of love … and keep going.

I did the unthinkable.

I stopped fighting the desires of my appetite and instead accepted what my body wanted. I began to eat anything and everything it craved, without reserve, assessment or analysis. Can you imagine the relief? I declared, from that moment on to never limit or manage my food in the name of weight again. My friend, I ate how Cheryl Strayed tells people to write: like 'mother-fucker.' Please don't get me wrong — I didn't start eating in a crazed get-me-the-hell-out-of-my-head way. No, I ate with clarity and dedication, all emotions in, with love, aliveness, and spirit. I started to respect the biological intelligence of my physical self. I found my intuition, long buried, long forgotten and which I had not since the age of about twelve trusted. Trusting, honoring, respecting my body and its desires became my work. I tasted my food. I noticed textures, flavors, and the beauty of what it provided: energy, sustenance, vitality. I vowed to always have enough food available so I could eat whatever my body wanted. I also learned to trust my old foe hunger. Do you get the magnitude of what I'm saying? Here's a thought to meditate on while you read — *what would it be like for you to completely trust your body?*

These life-changing choices, bundled together and practiced time and time and time again, spurred a new way of being in me. I came to realize I was acting — for the first time in my life — from self-love. I put down my weapons and picked up love. That shift is one I've never gotten over. It set in motion a chain reaction of choosing love over hate, which has seen all aspects of my life flourish.

While I ate in this new more nourishing way, I'd tell the voice in my head—The Resistance that wanted to keep me down at all costs—that it no longer held me hostage. I was done taking its advice about what I should and shouldn't eat. Slowly but surely, a strange thing happened. For the first time in twenty years, I experienced what it was like to not even think about food. The liberation of that feeling had me at hello. Only those of us who know what it's like to be out of control with our food can know the victory of that, right? I wasn't planning, analyzing, figuring out when, where, and how. When I stopped battling and started accepting, food obsession fell away.

As I take you on this journey of discovery, please know that replacing resistance with acceptance is not always an easy process to kick-start. From the outset, I had no idea how to even get to the start line. After milling about trying to figure out the how, I simply, consciously, declared I will. Back then, I didn't like my body and knew I couldn't pretend to either, but I did get that hating it was sucking the life from me. Confronting or confusing as it may be, if you find yourself in a similar position — wanting to accept but knowing you can't pretend to like your body, let alone love it — I urge you to declare peace and willingness now and simply start from there.

With my declaration in hand and desperate to start, but without a clue what to do, I randomly decided to stand naked in the mirror and connect, properly, with my physical self. I looked at each part of my unloved body in order to find something good, and then thank it. Can you

13

imagine how knee-crunchingly uncomfortable that was? My self-loathing filled its lungs and screamed at me but I stayed it out. You see, I really was ready to go to any length.

I looked past my inner voice throwing obscenities, hugged myself through soul-wrenching sobs and begged my body for forgiveness. I needed to make amends for the hatred, the shaming, the negativity stuck on repeat. I never knew before that moment what compassion for myself felt like. If you are yet to feel the wild-crazy goodness that self-compassion tows in its wake, I hope that day comes for you soon.

These early steps were profound and distinct from anything I'd done before. They put me in charge of my own well-being and self-acceptance was born. This new child in my life came holding a key that unlocked a door to a freedom I'd long since believed was possible. The kind of freedom that lets me follow my heart's desires.

So you can see, taking on these new, loving practices was a powerful start on the road to recovery. However, before you believe they were an overnight cure I want to make a few things clear: I didn't hate myself one day and feel blessed the next. I skidded and slipped, took two steps forward, tripped one step back, veered repeatedly off course. Yes, the journey was riddled with beautiful insights, but it included its fair share of tough lessons and hideous times.

As you recover your sense of self-worth and begin to accept your body, please give yourself the space to do it imperfectly. You'll have good days and bad days. You'll try things that work and things that don't. Staying with it, however it goes, and accepting all that is happening to you is one of the most powerful practices when it comes to living life on your own terms.

In 'Love Your Body, Change Your Life: Book One' (the first book in this series), I picked apart the different aspects of 'me' and mapped out how understanding these different perspectives creates a bedrock on which a strong recovery can be built. I learned I was more than the voice in my head that urged me to eat and the physical body I lived in. I was able to observe both of those and in the process of observing I found an abundance of personal power. This power allowed me to choose new thoughts, to watch emotions come and go (rather than be at their beck and call) and find peace in myself.

One of the main lessons I offer in Book One is how to observe The Resistance —that negative voice that pops up in our minds—and to live comfortably with it. At the end of that book, I promise that in this book I would take you, the reader, on a deeper journey beyond simple understanding, to the art of accepting, in order to open up a whole new vista of possibility for life.

If you are ready to kick obsessive eating to the curb, you are in the right place. If you want to follow a path that leads to the door of self-love, passion, personal power and knowing the awesomeness of who you are in this beautiful world, come with me now, I'll show you how.

What I'm Not Asking You to Do

Before you roll up your sleeves and accept everything about yourself and your life (won't that be something?)—I want to be very clear about what I am not asking you to do.

First up, I am not asking you to condone anything. This includes abuse, bullying, or harm you may have received. I am not asking you to minimize anything that causes you pain. I will be asking you to accept whatever has happened to you because it has happened, and also accept that it came with pain. Adding resistance to the pain (it shouldn't have happened) only adds more pain. In others words, I will be asking you to let go of resisting those things that happened (or are currently happening), not condone the fact that they did (or they are). Once you stop resisting, you stop dwelling. Once you stop dwelling, the power those events hold over your life will slip back a notch and allow you to take powerful action. As you will see, this will change your life in unexpected and beautiful ways.

Accepting things as they are doesn't mean I'm asking you to resign yourself to having the same life you currently experience with your food obsession, bingeing and purging without ever finding peace from it. As we go through this book, I will show you that acceptance of what is happening right now does not equal resignation that it cannot change. In fact, you will see that acceptance of the present is a powerful precursor to making positive changes in your life — particularly in the areas of your body and food.

Giving up on a dream because it is a long distance from where you currently are and you cannot see a path towards it, is resignation. Years of trying every means possible to get control over my food and failing repeatedly led me to believe I was holding onto an impossible dream. I became resigned about ever having the life I wanted to have, deep down. Even more scary, I gave up thinking I could make the contribution to the world I secretly wanted to make.

The way I now approach my dreams and visions and desires is vastly different to how it was when I was in the grip of bulimic hell. When I choose to go for something in life these days I make sure it lights me up in the present. I check my desires are not wishes conjured up to escape what I'm currently facing, but dreams that call me in a direction I'm proud to act toward in the now.

Please listen carefully: Acceptance of what is happening in your life right now will allow you to move toward a future that encompasses any possibility that lights *you* up. This is how it went for me and it's how it will go for you. When I accepted what was happening, I became unexpectedly free to move toward a different future. That is why I'm a big advocate for dreaming, exploring and picturing a world where you are thriving — including having a body you love. In other words, I suggest you imagine yourself living the life you have always wanted. However, I will also be asking you to deal with reality today.

Taking steps toward Radical Self-Acceptance could well take courage you don't know you have. It certainly did for me. I resisted accepting my life as it was for a long, painful time. I believed, wrongly, that acceptance would lead to more of the same; that acceptance meant giving up and giving in, having no hope to hold.

As you will soon see, it meant none of those.

In fact, quite the opposite occurred. It wasn't until I stopped pushing against the realities of my circumstances that I found the energy, power, and insight to create something different. When, indeed, I stopped feeling sorry for myself and turned that self-pity into self-love, the going in my life got good.

This turn in life is why I beat the drum of acceptance with gusto and persistence. I want that beat heard … everywhere. I want the rhythm of that knowledge to settle deep into the psyche of this world. Starting here and now.

On that note, let's talk about starting. There is never the

right time to start loving, accepting, and forgiving — or even a good time. There is only now. Please, if you take nothing else from my words: now is the time to start.

My Promise to You

"If you get the inside right,

the outside will fall into place."

~ *Eckhart Tolle*

As I said in *Book One*, I'm not a trained doctor, therapist, psychologist, counsellor, life coach, scientist, spiritual advisor, or biochemist. But I do know what it's like to be obsessed with food and then, remarkably, not to be. I have gone from every decision in my day being tainted with thoughts of eating, self-loathing and weight, to having space to build a creative career, be fully present and at peace in social situations involving food. I don't weigh myself, or plan what to eat or not to eat. I don't beat myself up about eating. I don't despair at my own thoughts. I fit into the same clothes year in, year out. Food doesn't dominate me anymore. I love my body and have gratitude for the life I live. I took a journey that brought me home to myself. In the process, I experienced profound healing.

Can I promise you will heal, too? Yes and no. From a scientific point of view, I don't have a randomized, double-blind, placebo-controlled, peer-reviewed, experiment to back up my theories. In fact, I'm not sure I can call my experience 'theories.' I only have my experience — what I have done and the results I got. I have read widely, enjoyed countless conversations and formed solid opinions about what works … for me. I have looked to spiritual sages and scientists to help understand why my practices may have helped. That said, because this book is non-scientific, I suggest you take my experience as a starting point — a way to frame the beginning of your own healing. Take what I say, try it on, change it up, and make it work … for you.

What I can say is that if you seek to find what works for you (and start by looking inward rather than outward to find freedom from food obsession)—you will find it. This is my promise to you.

When it comes to having the body you want, this second book will expand on what you learned in the first. My intention is that you find a deep sense of peace within. That peace can certainly begin by trying on the many cloaks of acceptance.

Chapter One:

The Paradox of Acceptance

"Understanding is the first step to acceptance,

and only with acceptance can there be recovery."

~ *J.K.Rowling*

As I said right at the start, I was slow to understand what real acceptance is. It is a distant shore from what I had previously thought. I'd read countless uplifting 'acceptance' quotes, nodding my head sagely. Next minute, I'd grumble about … something. I'd wax wisely to friends about the healing wonders of acceptance and yet I'd still focus on incessant irritations—my family wanting me to fit in at Christmas, the state of the art market, a health niggle, the friend who didn't invite me, the weather, the traffic… and on it went. Meh, meh, meh, these little internal conversations had nothing to do with acceptance. I hadn't yet moved from being able to intellectually get it (and seeing where others would do well to employ it), to letting it take root in the ground of my own life.

When I finally did allow acceptance to flourish, I noticed a shift in the way I interacted with the world. Bit by bit, instance by instance, I learned the intricacies, intimacies and realities of acceptance: where to look for it, how to implement it, what it feels like and how to keep going. I learned where I hadn't quite got to its heart; where I had imposed limits on it or made an attempt to accept, but really hadn't.

All of this learning added up over time to understanding that acceptance is a key ingredient in the recipe for personal power; one that cannot be left to the side, put in later, or substituted for something else. It's fundamental. Want to heal, transform or grow or change? You will need to get your head around acceptance and practice like your life depends on it. In any case, that is how the deal went for me.

When I finally turned my attention to this new realm, I discovered some not-so-nice things about myself. Turns out I believed myself entitled to things I felt that I, in particular, shouldn't have to work for. Without putting too fine a point on it, I was a first-class complainer. I had all manner of 'shoulds' and 'shouldn'ts' about how life was meant to roll out. I'd become a staunch advocate for fairness. Discontentment was my home base. All of which, without ever actually seeing it, kept me facing away from peace and, instead, trying to find tranquillity in six packs of chocolate muffins. When I discovered the true nature of acceptance, these things that had kept me stuck shimmered away, leaving a whole world of wonder in front of me.

I have already talked a bit about what acceptance isn't — condoning, minimizing, turning a blind eye, and my personal favorite, pretending everything is fine — so what *do* I mean when I talk about acceptance? Let's start by saying radical self-acceptance is less an intellectual grasp than a soul-deep, automatic way of being.

It includes:

1. Hearing The Resistance (the voice in your head that wants to keep you safe at all costs) at 3:00 am and listening with compassion but responding with stern authority: 'You may think it's important to wake me, dear Resistance, but I don't at this very minute need a list of why 'she' should be more grateful for my help. Go back to sleep.'

2. Being part of your soul's infinite healing system, rather than an ointment applied to a cut.

3. Practicing again and again. It's not a class you take, get graded for and move on. It's rather more like housework. Regular attention makes it easier to maintain.

4. Being an antidote to stress. As acceptance rises, stress falls away.

5. Seeing shame for your past wash away.

6. Not minding what happens in life. The way you *respond* to what happens is of way more interest to you than your circumstances.

Can we agree? This list is vastly different from the first one (minimize, pretend etc). One of the things you may notice is that every item on that list puts you in the driving seat of your life. That's because radical acceptance is about you having power over how your life goes — and leaving the necessity for others to change (so you can be okay) out of the picture. Don't underestimate the benefits of this when it comes to putting food obsession away for good.

It's now time to go a little deeper and shine a light on the paradox that acceptance presents us with.

The paradox, as you may now be starting to see, is this: anything we want to change by definition means we would like what we are experiencing to be different. Yet — and this is the kicker — in order to bring about change we have to be at total peace with how that thing is at the moment.

Awesome! If we want something to change we need not mind that it's happening. But isn't minding its happening fundamental to wanting it to be different? Isn't it the discomfort of the 'thing' that spurs us on? Well, yes and no.

The key to seeing how this works lies within the word 'minding.'

It took me years to get my head around what 'not minding' really meant. My lack of understanding was one of the main reasons my eating disorder stayed so firmly in place. I mistakenly thought that not minding I had bulimia was the same as not giving a toss. Not minding, as I now see it, is the direct opposite — it means caring deeply, but being okay that the experience is happening. It's making peace with it and knowing there is silver lining — a potential to grow and learn. Making peace with my eating disorder didn't mean I was indifferent to it or happy ignoring it. It sure as eggs didn't mean I could simply pretend it didn't exist and merrily dance off into the future. Not minding, as you shall see, is a whole different parcel of pomegranates to not caring.

Having declared that I *would* heal, I became fascinated with the paradox of acceptance. Wrestling with the idea (wanting something to change yet being at peace with it) became somewhat of an obsession — but this time, a healthy one. I have to confess that intellectually I didn't understand the paradox in its fullness until I had practical experience of how the equation worked. This entire book, in matter of fact, could be described as the story of how I went from powerfully resisting the things I didn't like in my life (and thus of course keeping them persisting) to making peace, finding power and creating change.

My first forays into acceptance were like learning to drive a stick shift: Jumpy, uncoordinated and slightly dangerous on the road, but I kept at it. You see, I really did want to be stubbornly glad about my body and everything else, I just had no clue as to *how* to practice acceptance. I found myself staring into the abyss of not knowing. It was at that point I realized: transcendence is going to take something rather radical.

Gaining insight in reality (rather than theory) of acceptance, I started noticing the way many self-help, personal development and spiritual texts often glossed over the importance of acceptance — if they mentioned it at all. Instead they dive straight into teaching how to use our imagination to direct life away from where it currently is: Don't like your financial situation? (or body, or relationship status), simply imagine an abundance of money (or see yourself as slim, or married) and those things, if you believe them strongly enough, will most surely come to you.

I can see why they do this. Acceptance is hard. It's gritty. It's painful. It's not a pleasant sell to say, "hey, there are external limitations you may never change (the basic shape of your body for example, or a disability you have.)" It's not exactly the stuff of inspiration to suggest that some circumstances may always persist (you may never get the financial freedom you so desire, or the slim body you so want) even though others have risen from the very same circumstances you are in now. Who wants to hear such dull news? The thing is, on the other side of that grim realization is the juice bar from heaven. Being able to look back at my years of out-of-controlness and know they are by and large a thing of the past — because I stopped minding — is worth every moment of discomfort.

That is why acceptance cannot be glossed over if you want to have long lasting inspiring personal power. Using your imagination — as shown in this book — is a beautiful, tremendously robust practice. But it's also one that will fall flat if you don't make room for acceptance *first*. Knowing that anything is possible is a life-altering concept, but only from the vantage point that your first priority is settling into the knowledge that you may never fully manifest your dreams. Living in the grand process of working toward something for the sheer delight of the journey (rather than trying to desperately escape how it currently is) is magic that I want you, along with everyone else on this planet to experience.

I'm asking you to keep this paradox in mind as you read on and begin to figure out acceptance for yourself. Hold true to the notion that bingeing, purging and self-hatred can be things of the past. Know that the way through them is by not minding they are there in the first place. That is a radical kind of self-acceptance.

In the following chapter I will take you through my many adventures into the realms of self-acceptance by looking at the very stuff of my life. As we look at each of the areas within I uncover, for your benefit, how practicing self-acceptance versus focusing solely on the changes I wanted to see, played out. I demonstrate how the power of imagination helped me make peace with where I was, and then reach into new areas.

In the final chapters, I suggest what you can look out for when it comes to acceptance, so you too can see resistance as a helpful signpost rather than a gremlin that runs havoc through your daily existence.

Let's dive right in with a story that begins in the sprawling city of LA.

Chapter Two:

The Stuff of Life

"These are the days that must happen to you."

~ Walt Whitman

Have you ever had a lightbulb moment? You know, the instant when an intellectual concept, suddenly, with high-density clarity, snaps itself into your bones. No longer do you simply understand, but you *know*. One of these moments struck when I looked at myself in the bathroom mirror in my small LA apartment. You'd be forgiven for thinking this particular realization would have struck a few years earlier, given all the personal 'work' I'd done - but there we have it. At the ripe age of thirty-seven, having understood for years I had a body *image* disorder as dysfunctional as my *eating* disorder, I had never so much as caught a glimpse of what that actually meant, like, in the reality of my day to day life. But just like that, I had it: I was disappointed in the body I saw in the mirror because it bore no resemblance to the body I wanted in my mind's eye. This gap — the one that hung between what I thought my body should look like and the reality of what faced me —was causing big problems.

To heal my eating disorder I had to heal my body image disorder. To do that I needed to mend the gap. I needed to be willing to turn away from the image I saw in my mind and face what I saw in the mirror with acceptance and love.

Holding a mental image of myself that made my heart sink was a crushingly bad use of my imagination. Getting this was a game changer. I was done attempting to shoehorn myself into something I wasn't. I was over waiting for my life to start once I got my body fixed. I needed a way of accessing the beauty of life (not to mention my thighs) right here, right now — not sometime down the track. It was time for my imagination to fuel my peace, not my grief.

At the time, when I noticed the gap and had the 'ah ha', I put pen to paper (as I tend to do) and noted what could be done. First was to accept that the image I saw in the mirror was not going to change in the next itty-bitty instant. Next was to swap out the vision of the body I wanted for one that served me better.

Before I swing into detailing the actions I took to change those images, let's circle back to the idea I raise in *'Book One'* about human potential and about taking steps toward any imagined future (which is always possible). There is a really important distinction to get here: On one hand, humans have the power to imagine any future for themselves and take a step towards it. It doesn't matter if that future is likely to happen. It doesn't matter if no one has ever achieved it before. What matters is that taking actions in line with that future lights you up. It also matters that the image you have of what you want to create is something you want to give your life to. The end game, in other words, is somewhat irrelevant — other than it creates enthusiasm and aliveness in the present.

On the other hand humans can hold mental pictures of things seemingly childlike to achieve. Losing ten pounds does not come over like a tall order. No one is going to look like you've just told them you're about to sell up, move to the desert and invent teleportation to Mars. But, when taking the actions toward that easy-to-achieve vision leaves you stuck, agitated, depressed, glum and reaching for the left-over lasagne even though you are so full you can barely move, it's time to re-think the vision and what we are giving our lives to.

This distinction falls right into the hands of the acceptance paradox.

One: If you are imagining yourself in the future as a way of escaping the present, no amount of visualization or imagination will make any difference. It will only depress you. When you are so out of cord with what is happening now, your imagination holds no power to help you create change in the future.

Two: As we've just seen, the pictures you choose to play of

yourself in your mind will either light you up or dull you down. To be clear, I'm not talking about these pictures giving you motivation or hope, I'm talking about how you respond to them emotionally.

Here's what I mean. For years I imagined myself stick thin, about twenty years old (no matter my current age), with narrow hips and firm bits that never wobbled. This picture didn't leave me feeling good about myself in the present. I'd have that vision, compare it to what I looked like now and feel like the world's biggest drop-kick. To comfort myself? Well, you know how that one goes.

The image I hold today is vastly different. The body I see is the one I have, not someone else's. I imagine it being able to move with ease and vitality. It is fit, full of life and energy. It desires nourishing food and stops wanting more when it's satisfied. I am my age. My hips are my hips. Things wobble and wrinkle and greys are emerging (in all sorts of places!). I am an average pear-shaped size, 175cm tall, with longish limbs, a shortish body, wide square shoulders, and skin that radiates health (thanks Nan, you rock). And that is about the sum of it.

This new and improved picture in my mind is a remarkable shift. I let go of my old depressing fantasy. Not because I believe the other vision I had for myself was impossible, but because it didn't leave me uplifted, like, right now in this life I'm living today. If it didn't cause excitement to rise in my blood and fill my heart with anticipation, I was throwing it out with the trash.

But let's go back to what I did before I created this better, more empowering vision.

At the very start, I looked to people who had a relationship with their body that I wanted to replicate. It wasn't the shape of their body, or how they looked that I was interested in, it was how they were in the world with themselves. And can you believe it? I couldn't find a single example of someone hating herself into success. There was no one I could point to and say, "see, she tortured herself into being a powerful, peaceful, relaxed human being, so how 'bout I keep on hating myself too." When I stopped and looked, the strong, powerful people I looked up to had a natural sense of self love. They were peaceful with where they were and then they took steps forward. There was no escaping from or fighting themselves, and they had no time for hatred.

I found myself writing this: My hateful means will never, in a million ugly years, take me away from where I am to where I wanted to be. Deprivation, punishment and shame will never result in positive change. My body cannot remain an enemy if I am to have the life I want.

And so it was. I took out a contract with me: from here on in I am learning and practicing self-love. That practice begins with accepting every square inch of my physical body is as it is — nothing more and nothing less.

Not knowing exactly how to go about finding self-love and accepting what I saw in the mirror, I simply did the first thing that came to mind — actually looking at and being with my body, in the same way I know how to be with a piece of art — notice, see, examine, just be with and get what you get. So I did.

The first time I stood naked and looked at myself properly, anger at the awfulness and unfairness of what I saw immediately stormed in. And what's more, when I thought about letting that rage go, I wasn't sure I wanted to. I mean, if I accepted this body and how I ate and what I thought and the disgusting things I did with food — if I truly accepted it all — I was pretty sure I was going to become everything I didn't want be. I would never, ever, stop eating. Food and weight would completely overtake me.

But, of course, they already had.

I had to stop and *feel* The Resistance that rose up at the thought of accepting my body. Dark, dense, emotion seemed to glare at me from all corners. To top it off, amongst the discomfort I could hear myself replaying an old favorite premise teasing me: "If you only looked better Emma, you'd feel better." The promise of that falsehood seemed so hopefully true.

Of course, The Resistance had relentlessly teased me with dizzyingly high promises for a skinny body. Happiness would arrive the day I got thin. Irritations would pass. People would love me. I'd be smarter and cooler and able to handle the stresses of the world. I'd do, be and have everything I'd always wanted.

That is the sneakiness of The Resistance. Not a minute before had I realized hatred would get me nowhere; that berating myself into submission would lead me back to exactly where I was.

As soon as I noticed that sneaky old replaying voice, I laughed. I actually guffawed out loud. I saw the quickness of its play. The way it nestled into a microscopic crack and started elbowing a deep dark canyon into my mind. 'Ah yes,' I thought, 'I've got your number.'

I got back to my body and being with it. I looked, I thanked, I noticed all it was and all it wasn't and promised to be loving from that moment on. And while I was at it, I promised to keep my word about this.

Being with my body as it was, was one thing. Making peace with everything I had done to that body was quite another. A niggle in the back of my mind started up, "sure, Emma, you've taken out a contract to get over this eating disorder and to learn to love yourself. But what about all the shit you've done. All the binges and vomiting and starving and exercising way beyond what's healthy. Really, you're going to say all of that is fine now?"

I didn't really know what to do with that niggling question. So I just kind of swept it to the back of my mind and kept focusing on being accepting of what I saw in the mirror.

And would you know, the very next day, with my new commitment to recovery, I went hiking with my friend Roberto where I learned the very practical difference between condoning and accepting. Sweating our way up the dusty tracks of LA's Griffith Park, we started discussing the inspiring lessons of Nelson Mandela. We were raving about his ability to forgive his jailers. We marvelled at how he accepted the way he was treated, but never condoned it, or even fought it. He didn't rile against it. He simply accepted it and sought to bring love to the situation. He forgave those who harmed him with compassion. He didn't seek retribution, he focused on the possibility of a better future, not a realignment of the past.

I literally stopped in my tracks. Unable to explain to Roberto exactly what I had understood for myself.

"What's got into you?" he asked.

"Nothing," I said and carried on.

But it was not nothing. It was just that I couldn't quite get the words out to express my insight. I suddenly got that I could forgive myself without condoning my behavior. I could see the goodness in myself and allow for mistakes. I could set myself free. *I could bloody well set myself free!*

For the rest of our hike, our conversation flowed back and forth like this:

Acceptance starts with love and allows for mistakes.

Condoning turns a blind eye.

Condoning pretends nothing happened.

Acceptance lives in the present and practices love.

Condoning says it's okay.

Acceptance says it happened.

Condoning feels hopeless.

Acceptance feels powerful.

Condoning is resignation.

Acceptance gets what is.

Acceptance is forgiveness.

And on we went.

From this conversation, I stepped away knowing that if Mandela can forgive his jailers, I can forgive myself. I can forgive The Resistance. I can forgive all those years of crazy eating. I can forgive the stuffing myself senseless then bringing it all back up. Yes, people, I learned a very personal lesson from a very great leader.

That night I was on a high. The power of forgiveness was in my heart, pumping the sweet hum of happiness through my veins.

In the course of the evening, I took a pen and paper (of course) and asked myself, "How do I keep practicing forgiveness? What can I do to make it practical and real? Is it enough to just say in my head, 'I forgive you,' or do I need to make more of a ceremony?" I certainly wanted my actions to speak as loud as my words.

My writing circled back to different aspects of myself and how I could use them to create a strong environment of forgiveness within myself. I stood as the 'me' that could observe myself and apologized to the 'me' that is my mind for all the critical observations I had made. I stood as the 'me' that had my best intentions at heart and forgave my physical body for not being what I thought it should be. In other words, I switched out different views of myself and took time to both apologize and forgive. I don't know if this is the right way to do this, but it worked.

That night I slept with the peace of a three-day-old baby. I ate an ordinary nourishing meal and felt entirely satisfied. I had taken one small step in the recovery of my eating disorder and one giant leap in personal power.

To solidify my forgiveness, I made a list of everything I could love about my body. I made the list real. I didn't say I love the way my legs look, because that didn't exactly ring true. I did say I love the way my legs work. I love that they can go hiking and run and ride a bike. I love that they are long. I love that they have held me up all these years. I love that they can wrap around a lover.

This acceptance business felt powerful. For the first time in my life, I got a taste of freedom from the revolving door that leads to bingeing. I felt relaxed in my own skin and saw myself taking strides toward increased vitality, a regular appetite, a body that is loved. I began to see why the big fuss about acceptance. I had inadvertently practiced the unavoidable, paradoxical, first step in making a significant life change by making peace with exactly how my body was, even though I saw a much better future for it.

In fact, I felt so good I thought I must be cured. Until a few days later, when I looked in a shop window and saw the ungainly size of my thighs. 'You are so fat,' the old voice started up.

Quickly pulled into the discomfort of that old voice, I found myself irritated at the thought of having to make peace with myself again. Seriously, again? Me? No! I've made my peace; I should be over this beating myself up business already.

Deflated, tense and in the grip of hateful thinking, I ate. I binged and felt the bliss of quiet inner solitude and then when it was over the regular gloomy pit of self-pity.

But I'd tasted the other side and wanted more of it. I wanted access to freedom on a regular basis. I reminded myself of the contract I'd made. I remembered Nelson

Mandela. I focused on acceptance and gave myself space to be imperfect.

And so, I got back to work. I got naked and stepped in front of the mirror. I cried. I became present to the life of hell dished up by that inner resistant voice.

As I was doing this work, a small inner whisper suggested I pretend to actually be Nelson Mandela. The Mandela Mantra became a kind of thing I did. It reminded to forgive. Then apologize. Forgive. Apologize. Seek to heal and seek to love.

In addition to this practice, I set out to create an acceptance habit. I scheduled forgiveness into my day. I read widely. I created a first-thing-upon-waking-manifesto: This day is the only one I have, exactly as it is. I can accept it, or I can wish it wasn't so.

In the same way that I understood hating the way my body looked was holding me back, I later began to understand hating the way my friends and family behaved was also keeping me down. Little did I know the chance to practice acceptance where others were concerned would present itself so fast.

Friends

When I arrived back in Wellington, fresh off the plane from LA—where I had declared to love myself—a group of close friends began acting in ways I didn't like. I found myself excluded, removed, or unwelcome in small and large ways: I'd hear of parties I didn't get invited to. A team of cyclists I'd competed with signed up for races without me. Trips away got organized, and I wasn't included. These friends were too busy to meet. Where I had once enjoyed a rich social life, I now spent many evenings and weekends alone.

This was not time for acceptance. These friends were being nasty, unfair and ruthless. I swilled about in a mess, bending the ear of any poor soul who dared to ask how I was.

Really, they were the ones who should change. They were wrong to treat me that way. How dare they. I was smarting and it was their fault. It was worse than breaking up with a boyfriend where at least a conversation might have been had. No one said, "Emma I'm breaking up with you." It just happened slowly, meanly, leaving me to figure it out.

No. This was most certainly no time for acceptance.

But of course, it was.

I didn't know how I was going to survive losing those friends. I sure as mustard didn't want to accept they no longer wanted me in their close circle.

Yet, dwelling on it was killing me. The mental space required to put forward my imaginary arguments was driving me batty. I stepped out of my mind for a moment and saw that not accepting their choices was leaving me unable to make good choices myself.

I got out the contract I made back in LA and knew that to honor it I'd have to make peace with my 'friend' situation. Continuing to not accept them would lead straight to the fridge, and was only going to forestall my pain.

My first job was to stop wanting/praying/wishing my friends were different. I had to surrender to the way they were.

Once I knew they weren't to be changed or fixed, my task became simple: feel the agony of losing something dear to me and then move on. I had to tend to my wounds. Having never been one to sit and be with intense emotions, here was my chance to practice.

I allowed myself to cry … properly. I stopped pretending I was above the hurt caused by playground antics. It took longer than expected, but I kept at it. I scheduled time to feel everything there was to feel. I brought curiosity to these sessions and used it for all it was worth. Taking notice of sensations plus the color, texture, and noise of this grief.

Then, one day, the hurt was gone. Its business done, it left. I was okay. In fact, I was better than okay. I was full. A sense of pride, excitement, and relief filled up the hole that grief had left. Life didn't look as scary and I didn't need food. That, guys, was big.

Not long after this revelation, I met one of those friends in the street and it didn't sting. In fact, I felt a little bad for her. She looked uncomfortable. I wanted to reassure her that I was okay. I wanted her to know I understood that sometimes friendships are done. It was not her responsibility to have my life work out. Yes, it was painful, but I learned a valuable lesson about myself and I was grateful for it.

In fact, I had taken a step toward accepting myself and the urge to binge was nowhere in sight.

Losing those friends and fully accepting it set me up perfectly for my next big lesson. One that involved a death, a will, and the dysfunction of a family.

Family

About a year after accepting my friends' choices, my Nan died. While she had played a small role in my life, I loved her dearly. To add drama to grief, a stereotypical family fight erupted over her final Will, that caused immediate clashing of horns between beneficiaries. The fighting disturbed me. It left me wishing for a different family, where old hurts were forgiven and empathy ruled the day. I hated the tension. I thought we were all behaving like spoilt, greedy children with our hands in a gold pot, bent out of shape that the Will didn't say quite what we thought it would.

I stepped onto my personal podium and judged my relatives with all the righteousness of an evangelical preacher. My family's disgraceful behavior became the starring role of my over-coffee discussions where I relished in describing a world of meanness, desperation, fibs and empire building inhabited by those I was unfortunately related to.

Acceptance? I don't think so.

As I wandered down this road of bitching and moaning, lolling in exasperation and irritation, I couldn't stop eating. I was baffled by how crazy my bingeing got at a time when I stood so virtuously in front of the others who were behaving so badly.

Are you beginning to see a pattern here?

Thankfully, that is exactly what I began to see. Again, my work was to revisit the pledge I made to myself back in LA — surrender to acceptance, and then hatch a plan.

As a small aside here, it's worth thinking about the idea of willingness for a moment. If I didn't have an eating disorder, perhaps I wouldn't have been willing to look more closely at what was going on. Perhaps I would have held on to my moral high ground and moved on from there — forever allowing the incidents surrounding my Nan's funeral to keep me well stocked in 'the terrible family I come from' stories to be wheeled out at dinner parties.

But I cannot afford such luxuries. I don't want to binge. I don't want to purge. I don't want to listen to the voice in my head telling me what rotten luck it was getting the family I did, and I certainly don't want to stand at the fridge hoping to find solace where it doesn't exist. All of which starts by taking the very first step: being willing.

Because I was willing and hungry for peace, I took a conscious, proverbial walk in my family's shoes to see if I could figure out why we were acting like we were.

I came to understand that my forbears are a deeply hurt people. Our family history involves broken promises, war scars, insufferable illnesses, secrets, and of course lies, along with fleeing countries (to follow unsanctioned love affairs and escape slighted lovers).

Probably not vastly different to the history of many families on this planet. But there I had it, right in front of me. And nowhere in this history did I see apologies from those who had hurt their relatives being handed down the line. There was only blame and justification. Not because these people of mine were bad eggs, but because that is what they had been taught from those who came before.

While metaphorically walking in my predecessors' shoes, the intention of my Nan's Will swam into uncomfortable focus. It had almost certainly been designed to cause trouble beyond the grave. Intending to embarrass, she did. The meanness of that saddened me. How awful for the ones receiving that slap. And how appropriate, I could now see, the behavior that followed. Compassion set up camp in my heart and down I climbed from the giddy heights of righteousness to a more level ground.

I stopped fighting against everything that was happening in our family and instead started looking at how I could offer love and acceptance.

When I think of it now with the benefit of years lived, I see the precious gift my Nan gave me: The opportunity to heal a family pain that had been kept alive for way too long. Unintentionally, she presented me with the perfect circumstances to grow, to learn, to put up my hand and say, "I'll take this on and help stop the ongoing hurt in its tracks." She didn't know I had an eating disorder, my Nan, but maybe she was smarter than I gave her credit for. Maybe she unconsciously knew that for things to change, they had to be bad enough for those affected to make an effort.

While I was living through this, an important point was not lost on me: I had way more tools and learning at my fingertips than any prior generation in our family. Mine was the first to enjoy mainstream access to personal growth ideas, like, we are not the content of our minds, or that the past does not need to dictate the future. We were the first to hear messages from great leaders such as Mandela, Mother Teresa, Gandhi and Martin Luther King as mere children. Expecting those who have had far less exposure to these ideas to heal the pain of their past is a bit like putting them in the cockpit of a 747, just because they have a driver's license, and expecting them to fly. This realization itself added to the acceptance I have of my family.

Before moving onto the connection between relationships, acceptance and transcendence, I want to make one final point about the connection between my family and my eating disorder. I don't like to admit it, but for most of my life I harbored a robust grudge against them. When everything else failed, they were to blame. I'd never have publicly admitted it. I was far too highly evolved for that (yeah, right). It was more like a last resort, in the safety of my own mind, when all other explanations failed. With hands in the air, flummoxed by why I was *still* scoffing behind closed door when I had so adamantly decided I was never going to again, I'd take out the I'm-from-a-dysfunctional-family argument and think, yep, it's all I have left, must be it.

When I think about how powerful it is to have the reins to my life in my own hands, I recognize the admirable job my parents did. "Thank you," I sometimes think, "for giving me everything you did, which allowed me to be the kind of person who can stand on her own two feet. For being someone who knows the buck of her life stops with her. For being able to grow and learn and take responsibility for getting up and getting on." Those have been the best lessons I ever learnt.

You may be wondering now whether I condone the way my family behaved at the times of my Nan's death. Did forgiveness cause me to find our actions excusable? No, I don't think our actions are excusable. It would have been much better if we didn't act like we did. I'm under no illusion that less pain would have been dished up if we had all behaved differently. But here's the thing — I now understand why we behaved as we did. And importantly, I understand we behaved as well as we knew how to. I don't for a second condone our behavior and I also don't have to broadcast it. I can accept we did what we did (within the confines of the information and circumstances of our lives) and find compassion.

These days, the minute I recognize my own reactions as justifiable and someone else's as a character fault, an alarm bell goes off—usually in the form of a desire to eat when

I'm not actually hungry. These tiny beautiful bells, I've come to see as divine wake-up calls. I ask myself, with a patient loving voice, "do I want to hand over responsibility for my life to someone else (by blaming them for my reaction to what is happening), or be a warrior for self-love and acceptance?"

This question is one that brings me to the next area in the stuff of my life that has helped me accept myself in a radical kind of way. This lesson took me on the biggest challenge of all, involving none other than relationships.

Relationships

I can point to the exact moment I leapt into a realm of acceptance that had the most profound effect on my life. From that particular moment, I never again questioned my self-worth. I never double-guessed if I had a fundamental flaw that everyone but me could see.

I had just moved north to live on a small island called Waiheke, off the coast of Auckland to take up a six-month artist in residence opportunity. The deal was that I got free board in exchange for three paintings from my latest collection. It was an amazing opportunity for any artist and one I jumped at. With no dependents and no responsibilities that I couldn't manage from afar, I packed my bags and off I went. I was on an adventure, had a clutch of new friends and was making a living as an artist. For all intents and purposes, life was grand.

Yet, in the background, as I was making progress in my recovery, I found myself still obsessing about food more than I wanted.

Yes, I had been practicing meditation while teasing out the different aspects of myself. Yes, I was proud at how I made peace with the friends I had lost and, yes, I was proud of the compassion I felt for my family.

Still.

I had an insistent nagging in my mind about being single. I was lonely and grieving the possibility of not having children—at thirty-nine I assumed that boat had sailed. Feeling rejected by society, I found it hard to take pleasure in other people meeting partners. The long empty nights alone rolled out like a sentence I'd been issued for my poor relationship skills and the grave mistakes I'd made along the way. I also couldn't shake the idea that my body, too, played its part in my eternal singleness.

While I was making peace with my body I would still look at the lumps, sags, and bits that wobbled and find myself thinking, "I can accept this is how I look, but who else in their right mind would want to spend their life looking at it?" In other words, while I was finding peace with and asking for forgiveness from my physical self, I still found it hard to imagine anyone actually finding me attractive.

When I stopped and listened carefully, I found The Resistance had taken a sneaky tack in its insistence at having me stay safe: It took the idea that being single was way safer — emotionally speaking — than being in a relationship *which might not work* and ran with it. To be fair, my family has a terrible marriage-working-out track record, which The Resistance bedded into my psyche and used for all it was worth. I'd seen a red carpet of pain roll out in front of the distress caused by marriages ending. The Resistance was not going to let me stick my hand in that meat grinder on her watch.

Analyzing these two things — one, blaming my body for my lack of suitors and two, a deep-seated skepticism of long term love — I could start to see as two sides of the same coin. If I could put to rest my unconscious reticence of long-term love, I could in turn stop blaming my body, and, if I stopped blaming my body, well, who knew what might happen? I got to work. I addressed the belief that any man worth his salt would naturally be repelled by me. The craftiness of this belief made me smile. Keeping that old chestnut roasting on the embers of my fear did a brilliant job at keeping me well back from long-term commitment. If no-one ever found me attractive, I'd never have to venture into a long term relationship or think about getting married, and then, I'd never have to deal with divorce. And divorce, from the perspective of keeping me out of harm's way, looked about as safe and pleasant as poking sharp sticks in my eyes.

Two things happened with this. I saw with twenty-twenty insight how well-honed The Resistance is at keeping me safe — she has zero, zip, nada regard for what I really want in my life. The Resistance is interested in one myopic outcome: having no shit happen, like, ever. Having me live a full and interesting life? Um, someone else's department entirely. In addition, I experienced a burst of mental clarity — if someone doesn't like what they see, it is their problem, not mine. I had, I must say, understood this concept intellectually at a much earlier date, but it wasn't until then that I got it in the marrow of my bones.

There I was, beginning to trust that a good man could actually find me attractive. Next cab off the rank was to deal with why I disliked being single as much as I did. Being single, after all, has nothing intrinsically wrong with it. In fact, it has some benefits I very nearly missed out on enjoying, even though I was single for the best part of fifteen years.

Over those fifteen years, I did my fair share of lamenting the absence of a matrimonial partner. And my dear friends (you guys, it's embarrassing how long it took me to get it!) did all they could to offer advice.

Many told me time and again that in order to find love I had to not want it. "As soon as you don't want a relationship," they would insist, "love will turn up." I'd want to smack them square in the face—"go back to your own smug life," I'd think, "you have no idea."

At the same time, their words plagued me. I'd lie in bed ruminating, "But I do want a relationship. Why should I have to not want one? They clearly wanted one. Otherwise, they would have stayed single. I have friends who really don't want a relationship, and guess what? They're single. Very happily single. I can't make myself not want one. I really can't, so basically I'm fucked. In fact, I don't ever want to not want one—relationships are great. I know loads of people who wanted a relationship before they had one." And onward that carousal would turn.

Never during this time do I remember luxuriating in the privileges that walk hand in hand with being on my own: always having music playing that I liked, furniture arranged exactly to my taste, nights out when it suited me. I didn't have to negotiate, or compromise … about anything. Now that I'm married, I wish I'd been more grateful. And in my desperation to meet someone, I almost missed appreciating that glorious slice of freedom entirely.

But I'm getting ahead of myself. I had to find acceptance of being single in order to find appreciation. And that only happened after I'd moved north to Waiheke Island to take up the artist in residence gig.

During my six months on Waiheke, I was part of a group art show in Auckland City. One evening, after we spent the day hanging our paintings, we, the artists, sat chatting, getting to know each other. The warmth of the conversation reflected the nature of the group. It was kind, helpful and fun. The discussion turned with ease towards how everyone met their partner — I was the only single one amongst us.

Normally in this kind of situation I'd have nipped straight down Sorry For Myself Street and silently started to justify why they were worthy of a relationship while itemizing all that was wrong with me. This time, however, I didn't do that. The Resistance (keeping me safe and single) was no longer raising its voice in my mind (and when it did I ignored it). I acted differently to my usual way of being and listened. Would you know, I actually heard what they had to say!

Each person described making peace with their situation by accepting it as it was. They talked about giving themselves love and kindness and enjoying the freedom that comes with being single (now there's a thought!). Each one had taken time to understand what it was they wanted in a partner and then patiently waited for that partner to arrive in their own time. Not one of them ever mentioned getting to a place of not wanting a relationship.

This is what my dear, earnest friends had been trying to tell me. They were not in fact saying I should stop wanting a partner. They were not even saying don't be open to one. They were trying to tell me to *not mind not having one* and then — and only then — to get clear about what next.

You could say they were telling me to put down the belief

that my life *shouldn't be like it is* and pick up on the beauty that *is already present*.

While it certainly seemed like fighting against my relationship status was the surest way to change it, my inability to make peace with where I was, was keeping me stuck. It was the overarching theme of my life that if I could just escape THIS (relationship status / body / the way friends were acting), then I would have THAT (happiness / peace / the fairy tale life). It-shouldn't-be-like-this was producing the show, and I couldn't get off the stage.

Charged up from the conversation with my fellow artists, I went home and wrote a list of everything I had to offer a man. For the first time in my life I felt as if having a partner was certainly possible (whereas before it seemed like an unattainable dream), and — most freeing and therefore importantly — that not having one was cool too. The excitement that arose from that understanding was palpable. I no longer 'needed' a man to make me whole or happy or have the life I always wanted. That, my friends, was already happening.

I got on with enjoying all that comes with being single.

This story, as you know, has a happy-ending. About six weeks after the exhibition (I told you I nearly missed out on appreciating life on my own!), I met the man I've been with ever since. About a month after meeting, I discovered I was pregnant with our daughter. We went on to have a son two years later and marry four years after that.

Please don't get me wrong. I'm not telling you this story to illustrate how I found a partner — I'm telling it to illustrate how I found acceptance. How I learned to go deeply into what 'is' and find the gift in it and allow what I am looking for to come to me in its own time, or not.

The beauty to me is this: had I not met Graeme (or another man), I would have been okay. I was not pretending to enjoy being single, I was skeleton-deep happy with it. In other words, I was poised to welcome a relationship into my life, but I didn't need one to be fulfilled or enthusiastic about life. This is the paradox at work. When I stopped minding the circumstances in my life, I was able to invite the change I had always wanted.

It's now time to switch tack and look at how to get out of our way. As we have seen in this chapter magic happens when we are willing to behold the stuff of our lives for everything they offer: Insights. Education. Growth. Goodness. The question I put to you now is this: Are you willing to get out of your own way and enjoy all that acceptance has to offer? If the answer is yes, let's move on to look at understanding how resignation, entitlement and complaining can wreak havoc in the pursuit of acceptance.

Chapter Three: Getting Out of Our Own Way

"We must be willing to let go of the life we have planned, so as to have the life that is waiting for us."

~ *Joseph Campbell*

Just in case you think I have this accepting thing one hundred percent nailed, let me tell you: No one is accepting all the time. Not me, not you. Probably not even the ones who look like they are. The relentless and famously difficult task for each of us is this: Get out of our own way, so if we fall off the wagon we have a way of hauling ourselves back on. Please remember: whenever shit goes wrong, the more awareness you have of your nature equals the bigger the problems you can tackle. That's because the more self-awareness you possess, the less likely you are to dive back into hating your body (or other unhelpful habits). And if you are anything like me, you know you have more to offer the world than fretting about the size and shape of your bum.

In a global sense, this chapter is dedicated to failure. We can go one of two ways when things go wobbly: We can give up, get resigned, feel hopeless and throw ourselves the biggest pity party on the planet. I used to be able to rustle up one of those on a dime back in the day. Or — and it really is a matter of choice here — grab hold of the lesson. Look at mistakes, fuck ups, humdinger ding-dongs, riding the embarrassment city bus and thank them. Get up, dust yourself off, remember we're human, remember we've got choices here people, and turn your slips and slides into gold.

When I find myself desperate to eat, to hide away, to find solace where it doesn't exist, or begin fantasizing about how much better life would be if I just lost a few pounds I can always (Every. Single. Damn. Time.) trace what is going on back to one of the following: Resignation, Entitlement, Complaining, Being Childish or resisting the fact that life involves eating Shit Sandwiches from time to time. Let's look at each one of these and how the very act of noticing them will hand us back the reins of our own personal power.

Resignation

Friends of mine recently signed up to run a half marathon and suggested I did too. When they told me their plan, I felt a familiar bubble of excitement. I'd had a hankering to start running again. A half marathon? Maybe now is my time. Planning out the potential 'whens' and 'wheres' of my training started occupying my thoughts. On the other hand, the list of excuses why *not* participate, started to surface. Back and forth I went.

This kind of mental tug-of-war used to plague me — way beyond its use-by date. I'd want something, but then not, then get all huffy and resigned about not being able to make a decision (hello hopeless loser me). But of course, I wouldn't stop there. I'd notch it up and start believing I'm a person who isn't up to much.

The thing is, I didn't see resignation as an inroad. I didn't see it as a gift and I didn't know what kinds of questions to ask myself to dust myself off.

These days I do, and I want you to too.

Here's what I did about the half marathon. I asked myself: "Is running something I really want?" Or — and this is the important part, the bit to be honest about — "is it a I-wish-I-could-make-myself kind of thing?" Did I really like the reality of what it would take? Did I really want to give five or six hours of an already full week to running? Or did I just like the idea of the end result? Yeah, in this case it was the later. I got all caught up in thinking I could be one of those sleek little running machines. And honestly, truly, really, I didn't want to put in the work; to do what it would take in that moment. Not only did I not want to do the half marathon, I wanted to stop pretending I might take up running some day in the future and put the whole thing to rest.

That decision was liberating. It was a good choice. I'd gone from hopeless resignation to liberation. See the gift in that?

Arianna Huffington in her book *Thrive* talks about unshackling ourselves from the things we keep on the back burner to be brought forward one day. For years, she told herself she would learn French and German and how to ski. When making room in her life for more freedom and peace (even those without eating disorders hanker for more personal power) she scrubbed everything that sat over her that added to her sense of resignation. In other words, she didn't have to do everything that looked interesting and she most certainly didn't have to be amazing, brilliant, the top of the pack at the things she did choose. The point being — neither do you or I. Sometimes the precise thing to do is tell that nagging 'ought-to' voice to back off, we are no longer interested.

On the other hand, sometimes those nagging thoughts call us and although they may seem impossible, they need a 'Yes! Let's bring this puppy home.'

My wardrobe, as an example, nagged at me for years. A longstanding resignation dogged me. I was uncomfortably caught between wanting a cupboard full of beautiful fabrics, clever designs and quality garments, and not having the income to satisfy my desire.

The gap between what I wanted and what I thought was possible was so vast I didn't believe I could bridge it. And yet, I didn't want to let it go either. My wardrobe desire was one I'd hankered for since childhood — but more to the point, having it work in the present inspired me. In this case, I was willing to give it time and energy. Spotting my resignation, I took action instead of dropping the whole thing. The wardrobe project was given the breath of life.

I made a pledge to love it. And while I was at it, committed to finding a way to have my long held desire fulfilled.

I started by finding the goodness that was already there and stopped looking for what was wrong. I enlisted a friend to help sort out what worked and what didn't with the clothes I already had, as my resignation had led me to keep items that didn't truly suit me.

I got clear about what I did want and began to relate to myself as someone with a wardrobe she loves as a work in progress, rather than a destination. I felt grateful for the clothes I already owned. I made a habit of scouring vintage stores and came home with bargains. I swapped clothes with friends and picked out things I'd get in the future when I had more to spend. To this day, this game is fun. Resignation is gone burger.

When you find yourself wondering around downtown 'Resignationville,' start by acknowledging you are there. Then be thankful. Like, "wow, okay gottcha, you have a gift for me you little beauty — you really shouldn't have, but go on, I know you always deliver." Try to access the two sides of your resignation — "I really want… but…."

Start, if you can (and remember to be super-gorgeous and gentle with yourself, the way a great teacher might be towards a remedial reading class) by accessing what feels beyond you. For example, when I imagined a massive wardrobe full of high-end brand names and bespoke runway pieces completely out of my budget, I felt despondent. Try to access, if you can, whether what you are chasing has an element you want now — in this current moment — or if it is just something you want in the future to escape what you are dealing with now. When it dawned on me that what I reeeeeally wanted was to feel excited when I opened my wardrobe door — and that there were a million ways to have that happen — I became enthusiastic. It got my juices flowing to think that every single item in my closet could fit and suit me. That getting dressed could be fun and easy. That I could enjoy the fabrics and the designs.

In other words, make sure that what you choose to spend time creating *serves* you. If you have wanted to be a ballerina for the last fifty years, please let go of any fantasy that doesn't make you want to dance, like right now, in your living room and pick up one that does. You may find that spending ten minutes every morning dancing your heart out adds way more excitement to your life than imagining yourself as the star of a ballet company. Accept where you are with your ability today. Then, take a step towards what your heart desires. Each small beautiful step will put space between you and resignation.

I'm happy to report that these days I have a respectful relationship with my dear friend Resignation. I trust her. She's a gem in the rough who makes my life sparkle beyond what I thought was possible. Even after all the attention I've piled onto my recovery, I can still wake up resigned about my body. And when I do, I don't mind, because I know that the path resignation steers me down leads to more peace, more freedom and more personal power.

Let's now turn our attention to a different beast. Similar in some ways to resignation, but a whole bunch more sneaky. One hell of a lot more dangerous. So slippery and snaky in fact, it's hard to grab, it's hard to see and to add insult to injury — almost impossible to acknowledge in oneself. But once again, as the deal normally goes round here, once you get the extent to which entitlement can sneer you in its grip, a different grip will loosen; the more you accept you've been acting entitled, the more food obsession will let go of you.

Entitled to What, You Might Ask

"Halloween is hardly what it could be.

Any other day of the year, hand a kid a chocolate bar and he'll be thrilled.

Do it on Halloween and it's worth almost nothing."

~ Seth Godin

I didn't understand how entitled I believed I was to the things I really wanted, but didn't have until I read a "Dear Sugar" advice column. It answered a question sent in by a writer who hadn't yet found success and was struggling to keep going. Sugar started by giving kind, insightful ideas about how to write regularly and how to take actions that could lead to the door of publishing acclaim that this young woman was so clearly committed to.

Then, bang.

She fired at a point that opened up a view of myself I'd never seen. Sugar simply said that *expectation* for success can only come from an unsavory sense of entitlement. It happens when we think we *deserve* the success we chase. It follows, doesn't it? When we think we deserve something, of course we expect it. Or — and this is even more insidious — we become cross, jealous and/or envious when someone else gets a result we are seeking for ourselves, by doing the same amount of work, or worse still, less. Oh boy, I was a master at comparing my successes with others. Right past go I'd proceed into those big emotions (jealousy, envy, anger) and head straight down big binge ally. While I had an inkling that making comparisons to others was a passport stamp to hideous island, I'd never caught sight of being entitled. That insight, you guys, has been massive.

But let's put jealousy and envy aside for a moment and go back to the finer points of entitlement. When we feel peeved, irritated, or downright angry that the end we desire has not materialized (as opposed to dusting ourselves off, realizing we can learn from our mistakes and moving forward) — part of us must, by definition, feel entitled.

Hell's teeth, I could hear myself think, I get irritated, peeved and angry when things I want don't materialize. I feel absolutely entitled to the things I want. When it comes to my body and eating habits, I'm like the kid in Seth Godin's quote above who hardly noticed the candy bar being offered at Halloween. My body is fit, whole, complete and yet I can't get past it not looking quite right. It's like the western world has declared 'success-Halloween' everyday about every aspect of our lives and we're all standing with our hands out. Successes have become like a right, and if not exactly a right, most certainly an expectation.

How on earth did all us smart, sensitive, well-meaning people get ourselves into this predicament? Where did we pick up this belief that we *should* be able to manifest what we want? The answer is an interesting one that I touch on in the next section. I look at the prevailing attitude ingrained in many of us that we can be, do, or have anything we set our hearts and minds to. But for now, let's focus on how to simply *notice* our sense of entitlement and what to do once we have.

Sugar, in her article, suggests that feeling so bad about not having something you want so badly is *only* possible if you feel entitled to that something. Said another way, we can be sure we've taken a big old spoon of entitlement if acceptance of our circumstances feels out of reach.

Those words shone an unimaginably, unavoidably bright light on all I believed life *should* be dishing out to me. All these years I had really truly believed I was born in the wrong body. Like really, THIS? So wrong in so many ways. And don't get me started on bulimia — I so did not *deserve* to have to deal with that. Seriously!

Sugar asked the woman to look and see if she believed that because she has been schooled in a certain way, enjoyed a certain level of access to things like education, money, and travel, it could be assumed her successes would be in line with those things. With stones falling in my heart, I saw that I certainly did. The column, as it happened, was not responding to a girl who came from a world of unusual financial abundance. She certainly didn't have it all, materially speaking, and clearly didn't always get whatever she asked for. This woman was a hard worker. She came from middle class nose-to-the-grindstone folks. But she had been brought up to believe she could be and have anything she wanted. And life wasn't offering the fruits of her desires.

Whoa. That was so ME. My parents in their utmost dedication to having me excel in whatever I wanted told me time and again that I could do, be or have whatever it was that mattered to me. As we will see in the next section, I took that to mean that whatever I wanted was a given and completely ignored the important distinction between what's *possible* and what's *definite*. Add to that my lack of dedication to the journey in relation to the end — I just wanted results, preferably yesterday.

But I haven't finished with Sugar yet. I felt she had heard the content of my thoughts and carefully crafted a letter to this young writer that would speak directly to what was holding me back. I stood stripped bare and yet, what she went on to say, magically, filled me with power.

Sugar asked the correspondent to stop being deserving and to instead be worthy.

Okay, now we are getting somewhere. I tried on being worthy and it left me on a different planet to being deserving. The latter left me fighting fruitlessly, the former accepting and at peace. 'Deserving' turns the future into a fix for the present. 'Worthy' makes the present an all-powerful place to be. See the difference there?

I took pen to paper and itemized the list of things I thought I deserved. This list was long. I started to note how different being worthy of the things on my list felt to being deserving. My world was shifting and I liked it.

Worthiness opened me up. Acceptance entered the picture and made herself comfortable. That's because you don't have to fight what it *is* to be worthy. On the other hand, Her Royal Highness The Duchess of Deserving insists we feel bad about our current situation in order to feel deserving of something else. She taunts us and teases us with the high hopes of a better end if we just rile against the present in her service. Goodbye dear Duchess, your reign is over.

As it is when you buy a new car and then see the very same car, like, everywhere, this exact thing happened to me with deserving and worthy. Talking with friends, platitudes on Facebook, marketing campaigns: Deserve was the main player and we were the pawns. Guys, there is a relentless conversation going on in our world called 'Life should be better than it is.' I've noticed the quick way we rally around each other and confirm our opinion, "oh yes, that certainly shouldn't have happened to you — you definitely deserve better, more, different." The sad thing about this is we inadvertently, in our efforts to be supportive and kind, gently steer people away from the place where they can deal with whatever it is they are dealing with. The here and now. We give such eagle-eyed focus to what we or our friends and family *should* be experiencing (a.k.a. are entitled to) we completely take our eye off being accepting. And acceptance as we know, is where the samurai sword of goodness lives.

But what about those things that really shouldn't have happened to us? The times when we were unimaginably hurt or wronged, abused, stolen from. The awful bad luck we had. The shitty way a family member treated us. The list of atrocities human beings endure is a long one. In particular, the atrocities at the hands of other humans. Saying we or our loved ones deserve better than what happened seems humane. It seems out and out wrong to suggest they did deserve what they got.

This brings us to an important point, one worth meditating on for a moment.

Shifting attention away from what *shouldn't* have happened to how we can powerfully react to what *has*, does not require a loss of compassion. By suggesting we stop talking about who deserves what, doesn't mean we believe people did deserve what happened to them. It's just not helpful to go there. Getting bogged down in what should and shouldn't be, takes away the gift of acceptance, wraps it up tightly, pops it on a high shelf and leaves it there, useless.

What I'm getting at here is paying close attention to how we *react* to our circumstances. Sugar's correspondent had no ability to react to her literary success (or lack thereof) powerfully because she was too busy being wrapped up in deserving her success. She was stewing about in wishing her world wasn't going the way it was and drowning in a big pool of hopeless. Sugar was offering a different way to react. One that pulled her out of that cesspool, dried her off and got her back to work. That's what I'm talking about.

Can you now start to see that when I suggest we throw out any mention of deservedness, I'm not suggesting we throw out compassion? Neither do I mean to encourage flippancy: "Oh, you had your leg crushed by a machine? Don't worry about it. Didn't you know you can react to your circumstances any way you like? Just look on the bright side." Umm... No. This is not what I imagine we replace the deserving conversation with when it comes to handling crappy circumstances.

Quite the opposite. I believe that without bringing in deservedness we can be *more* compassionate. Let's look at two very different scenarios. Imagine I've just told a friend I have bulimia, and I've had it for years. She starts down the, "oh, you so didn't deserve that in life" track.

"I know!!" I say. I like that she cares, but my heart drops. My mood darkens. I feel a little hopeless and depressed about the plight of my ways. My personal power has packed up and headed off to a tropical island to sip cocktails in the sun — no need for me here, I'll go lie on the beach.

In a different scenario, I tell a friend the same bulimia story. He says, "wow — I'm so sorry you had to deal with that, it must have sucked." Pause. "You are such a strong awesome person, so worthy of treating yourself with kindness and creating something better." I feel uplifted, empowered, full of energy. "Yeah," I think — "I'm not a loser who deserves better, I'm a good human being who is worthy of finding a path forward."

If you have suffered deeply at the hands of others or at the strange twist of unforeseen tragedies or if you have endured painful and dark times — I am sorry for your losses, hurts and scars. You are worthy of reacting to what has happened with perseverance and acceptance. Human beings have deep strength to draw on. And because you are reading this book, I know you are a human. All power to you, my friend.

While writing this chapter and having the 'worthy versus deserving' idea top of mind, the prevalence of the 'we deserve' platitude is not only widespread as I mention above, it's shocking. Almost every day, I hear a slant on the following:

I deserve a happy marriage.

I deserve a job I love.

I deserve better than this, dammit.

I've been hearing these things in the light of these

powerful entitlement ideas and in my mind I can't help but swap out deserving for worthy. Like this:

I am worthy of a happy marriage.

I am worthy of a job I love.

I am worthy of better than this, dammit.

A little ball of fire ignites in me every time I make this switch. It fuels a desire to accept myself. To be good to myself. To stand at the wheel of my own ship and steer her toward new, better shores.

Before we charge onto the next chapter about how visualization can help us get out of our own way (or, conversely, cause a big immovable road block) I want to tell you one more thing about the Dear Sugar letter.

The reason that particular letter made such an impact on me, was because after reading it I quit believing my body *should* look a certain way and that I somehow *deserved* all I wanted. Having the cost of fighting against how it *is* laid out for me so plainly (exactly zero ability to react to anything powerfully), I became willing to shift. I wanted peace and freedom — and letting go of 'should' and 'deserving' helped that happen.

Visualization

"Visualization works if you work hard.

That's the thing, you can't just visualize then go eat a sandwich."

~Jim Carrey

Okay. Let's go back to *why* we might feel entitled to the things we want. It's good to peek back sometimes and look at the why because it can help in the quest to get out of our own way. That said, *why* is not critical to finding personal power in the way that noticing *how* (irritated, stuck, like it shouldn't be this way) is. What I'm saying is, if the ideas in this chapter give you insight, great. If not, don't dwell here, focus instead on those areas that do make sense.

To see why we might be so entitled let's look back at some of the prevailing ideas of the last half of the last century. As a child born in the sixties, I was raised with the powerful belief that I was in charge of my own destiny. Whatever I wanted in life my parents made it clear they would support. I went on to read countless books suggesting if you can see it, you can achieve it. If you are positive enough, visualize enough and believe strongly enough, the universe will provide. Let me tell you — I loved this idea. I loved it because it kind of got me off the hook. I could spend hours imagining the thin, cellulite-free body, admired to kingdom come, with all my human pains far off in the distance, a thing of my uncomfortable past. It was a glorious belief that all I had to do was truly believe. But then, I'd skip right past the bit where you have to work hard, and rock on back to doing exactly what I had always done — despairing at the sight of myself in the mirror, feeling entitled to a body that wasn't materializing and complaining to myself about how bad it all was. I spent many an hour wondering why the universe wasn't doing its thing already!

The problem, you see, as Jim above points out, is that I'd visualize, believe, dream, imagine then head back to the same old sandwich. It took me a long, frustrating time to figure out where the power of visualization really lay. It wasn't that visualization is not a hugely powerful tool, it's that how to harness its power is often mis-represented. This happens in two ways:

1. When visualization is touted as a way to escape the present rather than bring peace to it.

2. When visualization is sold as the cause in the matter, rather than part of a bigger plan.

Let's look at each of these in turn, starting with using visualization to escape the present. You don't have to go far to get that most people seeking spiritual or personal development have a situation in their life they don't like; is uncomfortable, or is a barrier to living a more powerful life. Humans, by nature want to connect, to expand, to contribute. When these things are not happening it's a powerful motivator to seek assistance and get ideas about what to do.

Picking up this book, for instance, will be driven by your desire to end food obsession — because it's so damned time consuming. If you are anything like me, you would much rather give your attention and resources to making a difference in the world than to put on the gloves and go another round with the desire to eat.

As we know from understanding the paradox of acceptance, fighting against the present only perpetuates its existence. It follows then, that using visualization as a way to drag yourself out of your unfortunate circumstances is misguided. And worse still, as we've seen — when visualizing a future that makes you feel like shit about your current circumstances you will be less likely to accept them. Not helpful any which way you carve it.

This brings me to the second point — visualization being sold as *the* cause in the matter, rather than part of a bigger plan. Visualization is rather more like bringing a juicy steak to distract a dog while committing a burglary. It's a great tactic, but not the main attraction. How pointless would it be to buy steak and think the job is done? What about getting into the house, or understanding where the loot will be found? How about having a getaway route sorted? Sure, failing to distract the dog could scupper the whole thing, but the steak being the only necessary plan is laughable.

Visualization though is often sold as the main attraction. It's been held up as The Thing. We've got all excited about vision boards, hundred dollar bills taped to mirrors, imagining ourselves at the wheel of the car we want to own, repeating affirmations endlessly to ourselves, seeing ourselves thin, sleek and in charge of our destiny. And in all the excitement completely ignored the get-a-way plan.

Can you see what I'm getting at here? If you grew up in, or lived in the last few decades of the last century (in the western world) you will have been exposed to the opinion that you can be, do and have anything you put your mind to. You will almost certainly have been told that using your mind to imagine where you want to go is a direct ticket to the manifestation of all your dreams.

It's a much harder sell, and way less sexy to suggest that there are no guarantees for the manifestation of your dreams. Some people will succeed and some won't. What is a given is that you can take a step toward being, doing and having whatever your heart desires. Taking those steps, because you enjoy the journey, is where the juice of life lies.

Here is where I think the power of visualization comes in handy. It keeps your mind occupied, while you execute your master plan. It's not the main event and never will be. That said, just like the steak at the robbery, it's a brilliant addition to the toolbox for troublesome minds — and for that reason I like to use it. I have dogs in my mind and I do much better when they are distracted.

As well as tucking visualization away as a brilliant distraction technique, you may want to notice the kinds of things you see in your mind change as you develop a strong acceptance practice. Remember how I told you that when I got comfortable in my own skin an unexpected thing happened? That some of my old 'visions' that I had so desperately wanted didn't seem that interesting anymore? That I no longer wanted to look like a supermodel or felt desperate to be a certain shape, but instead wanted to feel good, treat myself well and move with ease and lightness? This is what happened when I started using my imagination to fuel my desire to enjoy the present, rather than escape to the future.

It's not that what I wanted was impossible or bad, it's just that when I stopped resisting the present, what I wanted turned out to be a different bag of turtles.

Complaining

When I was ten years old, I went on a school field trip to The Sir Edmund Hilary Adventure Camp. We did all sorts of scary and adventurous activities. There is one in particular that stays with me. I hung precariously over the top of a rock cliff, tied into a rope with a harness around my waist. The instructor told me to let go of him so that I'd be held by the rope and free to abseil down. My ten-year-old self kept trying to release his arm, but I couldn't. Finally, after much persuading, he forced me to let go. After a second of terror, I realized I was safe and free. I could descend the rock cliff in complete control.

While at first blush, this may seem an unlikely analogy to describe what giving up complaining might feel like (there is no obvious, scary cliff one is standing above when deciding to keep a complaint to oneself), the sense of personal accomplishment that rose up the moment my instructor let go has a similar pitch to the sense of freedom I get when I stop complaining.

Complaining, in its crazy-automatic, fly-below-the-radar-way is a powerful force because it provides a safe place to hide when the challenge of being responsible for how life goes feels overwhelming. You see, with every complaint issued, comes a one-way ticket to 'giveupville'. Because complaining, whether we like it or not, is only an option when we come face to face with a situation we don't like and believe we have no choices.

To understand how powerful it is to give up complaining let's look at what Tim Ferris of Four-Hour Workweek fame has to say about it. He became interested primarily as a fascinating thought experiment: Our words create our thoughts, our thoughts create our emotions, our emotions dictate how we experience our lives. If the words we start with are a complaint, well, you can see how that will end. He did a tally and noticed that thirty to forty percent of general conversation began with a complaint. Things like, "What the hell is this weather doing?" "What an ass he is." Etcetera. Having heard about the anti-complaint initiative of Will Bowen, a Kansas City minister, Ferris took it upon himself to do a twenty-one day anti-complaint challenge. It took Ferris three months to be able to go twenty-one days in a row.

In other words, to stop complaining is as hard as it is simple. When I tried, it was in fact, harder than I ever imagined (just like letting go of that arm all those years ago). Even today, with all I know about what complaining steals from me, I still, occasionally, find myself mid complaint. To make matters worse I get all jerky segues and pregnant pauses, stumbling halfway through sentences desperately seeking to rescue the conversation. The art of giving up complaints remains a work in progress. It hasn't been a once and for all deal. I hope, though, that one day it will be.

But let's circle back to Ferris for a moment. His definition of a complaint is a little narrower than Will Bowen's. Ferris's main interest in the challenge was to see if he could up his productivity. He was, it must be stated, blown away by the results — and this from a man who was already out of the park productive. Ferris suggests holding your tongue unless you can qualify how to rectify a situation that annoys you. Saying, "man the post office sucks," is out. But saying "man, the post office sucks at this time of day. From now on I'm only going to visit before 10am when the queues are shorter," is fine. And look, his definition is neither right or wrong. The important thing is to choose what works for you.

Bowen on the other hand suggests no gossiping, critizing or complaining. While Bowen's definition is a little more vague than Ferris's, it is the one I like and have adopted, for the following reasons.

When looking at complaints and what I wanted to transform, productivity wasn't my main concern. I had things like enthusiasm for life, being in my own driver's seat, providing fewer opportunities for the old 'you are fat and useless' thoughts to bump up against my life; those things. So for me, it was gossiping and complaining that I was — and still am — out to oust.

To this day, I'm yet to go the full twenty-one days. As I said, it's a work in progress which I start and start again. It is tempting to ignore my small transgressions — ones like laughing at a mean comment that rings true. Or telling a story where I got hurt but focusing solely on the shortcomings of another person. The reason I keep at this challenge, is that I know well enough, every time I break the run, there is fall out. Usually small, but there nonetheless: I find myself reaching for another cookie after the enjoyment of eating has gone. The Resistance pipes up and I find it hard to ignore her. I wake at three in the morning feeling frightened of the world and can't quite put my finger on why.

Being conscious of complaining is a great mindset to take with you into the next chapter, where we look at the enlightening distinction between being childish and childlike.

Childlike vs. Childish

In her book *Big Magic*, Elizabeth Gilbert recommends approaching art with a childlike frame of mind. This idea is neither original nor surprising — the artist as an innocent is an age-old concept. What got my attention, however, was when she recommended vigilance about being childlike as opposed to being childish. Being childlike brings a sense of wonder about what might be possible. It opens us up to curiosity and inquisitiveness. Being childish, on the other hand, kills creativity. When we throw tantrums, get demanding or act petulant, we are being childish. And human beings, as Gilbert points out, cannot rise to great creative expression when they are being childish.

I read *Big Magic* with my writer's hat on, seeing where I might deepen my own creativity (a topic I'm endlessly interested in) and found myself delighted at how this lesson could be applied to any number of things. It struck me, in particular, as relevant to how I approach my obsessiveness with food.

When I look at my life through the lens of being childlike, I feel free to explore how I approach food and deal with emotions. I become observant, curious, and open to wonder. These are delightful ways to relate to the world around me. Can you start to see the possibility of this for yourself? When I'm being childish, on the other hand, I'm easily disgruntled. I can see that while I enjoy spending blissful minutes imagining a better future (a clearly childlike state), flicking the switch into churlish abdication of responsibility for being present and accepting (hello childishness) can happen in the blink of an eye. Being aware of the two child states (childlike and childish) has allowed me to notice that switch getting activated and to step back for a moment. What's more, it has helped me welcome inevitable obstacles that arise in day-to-day living and dance with them.

Day to day obstacles, indeed, are the subject of the next section. When we are unwilling to accept obstacles that arise, we — of course — have a problem. Mark Manson has a unique view on this called, 'eating the shit sandwich.'

Acceptance and 'The Shit Sandwich'

"Everything sucks, some of the time."

~ *Mark Manson*

Reading a ten minute article by Mark Manson changed my life. He argues that life is not sunshine and roses everyday and that this is a good thing. I actually found myself thinking, "brilliant. Bring on the crap."

Not only had I been approaching obstacles in my life like they had to be overcome, but somewhere along the way I came to believe that my personal development quest was to get everything perfect. You know, like all problems solved, all challenges conquered, all imperfections ironed out — at which point I'd be the happy, skinny, successful, brilliant, wealthy, married, world-saving person that I always knew I was and sit back to enjoy the sunset years of my life, with servants catering to every vegan need in my glorious mountain house, divinely decorated with beautiful and timeless objects of desire.

Okay, so I may be overstating the pursuit of my fantasy with a bit of dramatic license. The point is, on the one hand I knew that the fantastical place I was trying to get to was an imaginary nirvana. I also couldn't get past trying to fix the things in my world that I thought were wrong.

As each word in Manson's article sank into my already plummeting guts, I grasped the extent to which I believed I could get to a place where I'd be happy all the time. So, you see, each and every time I wasn't satisfied, or failed to rise to a challenge powerfully, or didn't like what was happening in my life, it was a problem. I'd get stuck, unable to let discomfort, down days, or circumstances that I didn't like simply pass by.

Manson's article gave me permission to relax. He pointed out that with every choice to swing for something, anything, comes its own particular side of shit sandwich. Want to be a doctor? You'll be dished up ten years of relentlessly brutal schooling. Want to be a parent? Sleeplessness will be on your plate. Want to be an artist? Prepare yourself for hundreds, if not thousands of rejections, criticisms and slaps in the face.

In other words, nothing is ever relentlessly pleasurable, exciting, or fabulous. As Manson states so economically above, "everything sucks, some of the time."

It's worth poking a stick at this a little bit, given the pervasive wisdom that 'when you embrace a decision that is right for you, the universe will rise up to meet you.' It's only too easy to imagine that the path towards said decision will be smooth and easy. That troubled waters —

because a decision is 'right' — will be nowhere in sight. This logical leap, while easily made, does nothing but distract us from the goodness in life.

Like, for example, last year, my husband and I decided to sell our house and build a new home. The decision took years to arrive at. Once made, however, was clearly a choice that would benefit us. Many things fell pleasantly into place. On the other hand, many things didn't. I hadn't planned for the stress heaped onto our relationship that moving house with two small children while he worked himself near into the ground would have. Living with all our stuff jammed into a house half the size of our previous one wasn't easy or fun. Neither did I plan on a hormonal shift hitting me (hello peri-menopause, you little devil you) that would require dealing with mood swings, heat management and, I'll say it, bursts of irrational indignation. It was easy to wonder if the decision to uproot ourselves and build a new house was the right one. Had the universe really come up to meet us? Looking through the lens that 'good' choices are ones that are devoid of hardship would have encouraged us to throw the baby out with the proverbial bathwater. But understanding 'shit sandwiches' are a side dish to any choice makes riding the bumps of life a million times easier.

In other words, the worst thing we can do is think the choices we make won't suck sometimes. That we will be spared hardship, boredom, loneliness, criticism, failure, or challenge. Please be very careful when looking at examples of people who have made similar choices to you and not had to deal with some flavor of shit sandwich. Some parents have children that sleep through from three weeks and never experience sleep deprivation. Some actors get their break at six years old and never have to wait tables. These examples are the exception, not the rule. They tease us and taunt us with the 'see-it's-possible' mantra. But they do nothing to help us get comfy with allowing the sucky times that we might be dealing with to pass.

When I think about my journey from bulimic hell to a body I love, I can see I had expected to be in the clear when it came to challenges, because my decision was one that would clearly improve my life. Time and again I'd be surprised that life was dealing cards I didn't like. I wanted to be the exception, not the rule, in my healing. I wanted to the be one that made a contract with herself to heal and then never again have an urge to eat, a bad thought about her body, or be overcome by a fit of self-disgust. This fantasy did nothing but keep me in the hard clutches of non-acceptance. Non-acceptance, in turn, made healing harder to grasp.

These days, thanks to Mr. Manson, I'm way quicker to accept that a challenge is just a natural part of life. That some days I wake up grumpy, bored or irritated by the size of my thighs. I let those days pass. I don't for a second let them elbow their way in to knowing I have made huge inroads into my healing.

Chapter Four:

Onward

"Acceptance is a small quiet room."

~ *Cheryl Strayed*

Every year over the past ten, I have thought about telling the story of how I went from bulimic torture to a body I love. Not because I wanted to help others, (I had enough on my plate just helping myself!) or even because I wanted more love in the world and less shame, which, believe me, I do. You see, I simply wanted to be authentic and have no secrets between me and the world.

The call to tell the story of my own transcendence got so forceful, it became physically uncomfortable not to heed it. On top of that, when I saw new diets and nutritional programs and healthy eating plans being sold as if they would solve the problems of overeating, I'd wish a better conversation could rise above their inaccurate promises.

But …

Instead of taking action, I'd only reach as far as imagining myself telling the story of how I dismantled my shame and being trapped in a body I hated.

I never quite got the courage to speak out.

Until …

In 2014, following the death of Robin Williams, I was moved by the attention mental illness was getting in the media and pleased by how far society had come. I found myself wishing I had bipolar disease instead of bulimia. The acceptance of the fact that depression is an illness seemed so liberating. When I pulled back though, and saw the folly in that wish, I realized what I really wanted was a world where I didn't feel so ashamed to have the condition I had. It was time to put my hand up.

Thinking that perhaps a good place to begin would be to start a conversation to strip back some of the misbeliefs about bulimia, I wrote a blog post admitting I was bulimic and had been for twenty-five odd years. With courage, I didn't know I had, I pushed "publish" and the world never looked the same. My bravery instantly dissolved into regret. Dismantling the internet so no one could read what I'd written seemed like a good plan. For the first twenty-four hours, I couldn't leave my house. I was positive everyone would be snickering and talking in excited tones about what a loser I was. I stopped opening my email or checking my phone. The idea that those who held me in esteem might understand the realness of my life was too much.

When I did muster the courage to read my mail, go shopping, open my door, I was shocked by the love. Beautiful, moving, soul-baring messages poured in. Many from friends and acquaintances I had known for years, who had lives that, unbeknownst to me, paralleled mine.

A few weeks down the road it hit me: I didn't only survive doing something so scary, I had become stronger. A layer of shame had washed right off.

It took all those years to be that open for one reason and one reason only: I still hadn't fully accepted myself. Not entirely, like stand in front of a crowded room and say, "this is what it's like in the recesses of my quiet self. This is what I did and I am shamelessly proud of myself, anyway. Not just the recovery bit, or the success story that demonstrates from here to there, but also of the girl who spent years travelling the world shoving her fingers down her throat trying to get thinner so that life would be bearable." Yes, dear reader, I am proud of her too.

It wasn't until I spoke up and spoke out that I totally understood the starring role that acceptance played in my overall recovery. Acceptance had featured in that major sense of telling the world, but also in each small, beautiful, not so obvious, step along the way.

As you have read this book I hope you, too, have dug more deeply into your own journey with acceptance. I don't mean I hope you've rushed out and started a blog (unless that's your gig) to tell the world your innermost shame. I do hope though, you've come to terms with all that you are and love yourself as a whole person who doesn't need to be fixed. It means you will settle into a place where shame no longer resides in the creases of your being. That you find compassion, forgiveness and love for your circumstances, mistakes, body and all that has and hasn't happened to you.

With the perspective that a few years has given me, I can see that the longer I sit on the bus of acceptance, the more it delivers me to where I always want to be—past obsession, food management and relentless, fruitless attempts to escape a body I didn't like — to a new place steeped in freedom and peace. This has turned out to be the life I always wanted — I just couldn't ever find the door in.

Perspective has also provided me with insight into my own capabilities. I didn't know before practicing radical self-acceptance that I might be up to a job I secretly hankered for — creating something of value and beauty that might touch the hearts of other people.

And of course, lest I forget, having self-acceptance doesn't mean every moment of my life is spiced with blissful joy. I still have problems to solve, challenges to face, circumstances that press me into corners I do not like. My problems, though, are better ones and the good times of my life outweigh the bad. I don't feel helpless or hopeless.

I feel empowered and alive.

Yes, acceptance leads to a good place, but it hasn't lead to cymbals resounding as I'm lifted up to celebrate my contribution to humanity. We are all adults here, and this is not a fairy tale. Acceptance is more solid and more subtle than those fantasies. What I want you to remember is this: If you accept everything about yourself, you will feel the sublime peace of being okay in your own skin. You will be able to look in the mirror and know shameless love in the eyes that greet you. You will be open enough with your secrets to know there is at least one more person (you!) in the world who is turning towards love and away from shame.

Acceptance, as Strayed so eloquently tells us, is more like "a small quiet room." It's a room I seek out regularly and I hope you will too.

Practicing

It's not overstating it to say that in acceptance I have found transcendence. Transcendence from a world of obsession to a life of not minding. As we have discovered, acceptance is not something to be learnt, done, and put away. It's not a model to be built and admired in its perfection. It requires ongoing awareness and maintenance. In other words, it's about learning to see the signposts that indicate it's time to start accepting so you can put your energy into better pursuits. These signposts are far more obvious when acceptance is practiced on a regular basis.

My practices look like this:

1. Notice what I am resisting.

2. Forgive everything and everyone, including myself.

3. Find compassion.

About once a month, I write at the top of a blank page, 'Things That Shouldn't Be Like They Are.'

As I write, I make sure I note everything I've been complaining about. Like the weather; an aspect of my children's school; the state of my house; the state of my business, our finances, my wardrobe. Anything that I've found myself saying "man, seriously, it's crazy, or fucked up," or any way I've found to say something shouldn't really be like it is.

I go through each complaint and put a ring around it and then look to see what it is I'm resisting. For example, the weather is just the weather; I can't do anything but fully be with how it is. Once I remember I am powerless over the weather (but in full control over my reaction to it), I am reacquainted with its beauty. I can feel its energy. I can see the light changes, the color changes, the force of it, the power it offers us. The same goes for the people in our lives. Once we stop trying to change a person we are more open to seeing the goodness in them.

I ask myself if I feel entitled to something I don't have. Do I believe I deserve something different? Am I willing to do what it takes to have the thing I am wanting and can I find a sense of worthiness to take action? Please remember, these 'entitlements' are the hardest things to see, but hold the most potential for change once recognized.

I make a point of adding to my list those people who have wronged me. I take a minute to see the world from their perspective and understand why they might be acting the way they are. I look to see if they need an apology from me for judging them harshly, or for behaving towards them in a way that only keeps the bad blood flowing.

I remind myself, when attempting forgiveness, that compassion has nothing to do with condoning hurtful behavior, or minimizing the impact it has. And remind myself of the ability I have to respond to circumstances in a way that best serves me and others. Feeling angry, annoyed, resentful, bitchy, hard done by or irritated does not leave my life turning out the way I want it to. In other words, it's worth the effort to get to compassion and go from there.

If I've been particularly bopped about by The Resistance (you know how that goes), I simply spend ten minutes or so breathing in, focusing as much as I can on my breath and the sensations around me, with an offer of acceptance to myself on the out breath. What I do is feel my breath going in to my lungs as I breath in and then I say the word 'acceptance' to myself on the out breath. As I do this, I begin to feel calmer, freer, more peaceful.

Practices Continued

"Owning our story and loving ourselves through that process is the bravest thing that we will ever do."

~Brene Brown

Today I commit to the following practices:

1. Declaring myself to be someone who accepts all there is to accept.

2. Looking at myself in the mirror on a regular basis and thanking my body for its service.

3. Forgiving and accepting others: Seeking to be compassionate and reminding myself that everyone is doing the best they know how with the information they have. I am not in their shoes and cannot judge accurately. Reminding myself that compassion has nothing to do with condoning or minimizing the impact of someone's behavior, but that compassion will place both of us in the best place to heal.

4. Inviting slow healing breaths on a regular basis, to experience acceptance inside and out.

5. Unearthing entitlement: Writing in my journal (or whatever works best) to see where I have fallen into the trap of thinking I'm entitled to something.

6. Noting everything I think shouldn't be how it is and allowing it to be, without slipping into feeling resigned or resentful. Allowing all to be as it is while noticing the gap between what is and what I want to be without resignation or complaint.

In addition to the above practices, be prepared to work on their design. Create them to work for you. Make it your mission to seek acceptance and to create real, in-your-world structures to assist you in that process.

Chapter five:
'Til We Meet Again

"Weight loss does not make people happy, or peaceful. Being thin does not address the emptiness that has no shape or weight or name. Even a wildly successful diet is a colossal failure because inside the new body is the same sinking heart."

~ *Geneen Roth*

I started this book by saying I used to think bulimia was the worst thing ever. It took me years to understand bulimia was the connection between my sinking heart and the way I felt about my body. Partly because of the incessant media bombardment that told me being slimmer, fitter, healthier, bendier, darker, lighter or slightly rearranged in some way would lead to all the happiness I wanted falling at my door. It is no wonder I kept thinking that if I just got my body in shape everything else would follow. It's easy to see why I kept trying to manage my food and weight even though the things I did never resulted in what I really wanted — a new me.

How I came to transcend the grip that food had on me has been a multi-faceted process. It wasn't a one hit deal and it certainly didn't happen overnight. Even after I understood who I was, as told in *Book One*, and came to accept everything about myself and my life as detailed in this book, I still had to deal with what I put in my mouth. How I learned to follow the call of my appetite, my emotions and my joy (and never let anyone tell me what to eat or not) is the subject of Book Three in this series—*Eat Like A Motherfucker*.

The work I suggest doing in the pages of my books takes grit, commitment and stepping out to the flimsy outskirts of life. Although the air is rich and the view is magnificent out there, it can feel precarious at times. Each step you take towards knowing who you are, accepting yourself and next, getting ready to eat in an entirely new way, will help you know yourself to be the human being you always knew you were.

It is my hope that as you read my books, you will no longer seek to find a better tomorrow in the food you eat today; that you can leave the false promise of diets and weight management regimes behind. I want you to unveil the enormous potential of yourself and rethink what is possible for your life, your body, and the way you eat.

To deepen your healing, please come join me again soon.

****

Stay In The Loop

If you would like to know when Book Three (Eat Like A MoFo) in the *Love Your Body, Change Your Life* series, and other titles, are published — sign up to my readers group/newsletter at emmawright.co.nz

If reading this book made a difference to you, there are two ways you can help others to find it.

First: Amazon reviews are invaluable. If this book made an impression — for better or worse — please leave a review).

Second: You can recommend this book to friends who might like/value/appreciate it - word of mouth is the best kind of validation.

If you want to say Hi, or have any questions, email me at emma@emmawright.co.nz

To check out my blog and latest projects go to emmawright.co.nz

About Emma

When I was thirty-seven, I forgave myself for having an eating disorder and for being single and childless.

In that moment, I also found out who I was.

I knew right then that I (like you and everyone on the planet) have great personal power, but often fail to use it.

Self-love changed the course of my life, healed my wounds, empowered those around me and transformed the world I live in.

It all depended on one thing: being ready to surrender.

I have devoted my life to understanding how human beings operate — and how we can be more fully ourselves.

There is always more to learn.

My Work & Career

I am the author of three books (so far). Book One in the *Love Your Body, Change Your Life* series and *Feel Good Friday: 40 Unexpected Ways To Feel Good About Your Life* and, of course, this one.

I have sold over 500 paintings to clients all over the world.

I've been profiled in magazines and newspapers in four different countries.

I've have supported myself with my creativity for over ten years.

I have been called "brilliant" and "wise" by some; "rude" and "unoriginal" by others.

It's been an eye-opening road.

It all started in front of a mirror uttering the words, "Emma I forgive…" and a bucket full of tears.

Other Bits & Bobs

I was born in Auckland, New Zealand. I currently live in the beautiful leafy South Island village of Arrowtown with my husband and our two children. My favorite human is Sai Maa. My favorite poet is Rudyard Kipling. My favorite spiritual leader is Eckhart Tolle. At one point in my life, I was a brand consultant for a graphic design agency. I love sunsets, all kinds of books (from literary to spiritual, biography to business non-fiction), coffee, movies, fashion, skiing, mountain biking, swimming with my children, and of course, any opportunity to write, converse, create and grow.

In addition, I am much happier since turning 40. Forgiveness is beautiful.

For now, I reckon that's all you need to know.

Printed in Great Britain
by Amazon